# Adult Scoliosis

A Beginner's 2-Week Quick Start Guide on Managing Adult Scoliosis Through Diet and Other Natural Methods, With Sample Recipes and a Meal Plan

mf

copyright © 2022 Patrick Marshwell

All rights reserved No part of this book may be reproduced, or stored in a retrieval system, or transmitted in any form or by any means, electronic, mechanical, photocopying, recording, or otherwise, without express written permission of the publisher.

# Disclaimer

By reading this disclaimer, you are accepting the terms of the disclaimer in full. If you disagree with this disclaimer, please do not read the guide.

All of the content within this guide is provided for informational and educational purposes only, and should not be accepted as independent medical or other professional advice. The author is not a doctor, physician, nurse, mental health provider, or registered nutritionist/dietician. Therefore, using and reading this guide does not establish any form of a physician-patient relationship.

Always consult with a physician or another qualified health provider with any issues or questions you might have regarding any sort of medical condition. Do not ever disregard any qualified professional medical advice or delay seeking that advice because of anything you have read in this guide. The information in this guide is not intended to be any sort of medical advice and should not be used in lieu of any medical advice by a licensed and qualified medical professional.

The information in this guide has been compiled from a variety of known sources. However, the author cannot attest to or guarantee the accuracy of each source and thus should not be held liable for any errors or omissions.

You acknowledge that the publisher of this guide will not be held liable for any loss or damage of any kind incurred as a result of this guide or the reliance on any information provided within this guide. You acknowledge and agree that you assume all risk and responsibility for any action you undertake in response to the information in this guide.

Using this guide does not guarantee any particular result (e.g., weight loss or a cure). By reading this guide, you acknowledge that there are no guarantees to any specific outcome or results you can expect.

All product names, diet plans, or names used in this guide are for identification purposes only and are the property of their respective owners. The use of these names does not imply endorsement. All other trademarks cited herein are the property of their respective owners.

Where applicable, this guide is not intended to be a substitute for the original work of this diet plan and is, at most, a supplement to the original work for this diet plan and never a direct substitute. This guide is a personal expression of the facts of that diet plan.

Where applicable, persons shown in the cover images are stock photography models and the publisher has obtained the rights to use the images through license agreements with third-party stock image companies.

# Table of Contents

**Introduction**   7
**What Is Adult Scoliosis?**   9
    Symptoms   12
    Causes   13
    Risk Factors for Developing Scoliosis   14
    Prevention   15
    Diagnosis   15
    Treatment for Scoliosis   17
**Psychological and Emotional Impact of Scoliosis**   20
    Mental Health Challenges Faced by Scoliosis Patients   20
    Strategies for Emotional Well-Being   22
**Natural Methods to Manage Adult Scoliosis**   25
    Exercise   25
    Chiropractic Care   27
    Massage Therapy   28
    Acupuncture   29
    Herbal Medicine   30
**Daily Living with Scoliosis**   31
    Ergonomics Tips for Scoliosis   31
    Helpful Daily Aids   32
    Scoliosis-Specific Exercise Programs   34
**Technological and Medical Advances in Scoliosis Management**   41
    Advancements in Non-Invasive Diagnostics   41
    Minimally Invasive Treatments   43
    Emerging Therapies and Technologies   44
**Case Studies and Success Stories**   47
    Support Systems for Scoliosis Patients and Caregivers   49
**Managing Adult Scoliosis Through Diet**   53

|  |  |
|---|---|
| List of Foods to Consume | 53 |
| List of Foods to Avoid | 56 |
| **Weekly Meal Plan** | **59** |
| **Sample Recipes** | **61** |
| Salmon Wrapped in Bacon | 62 |
| Baked Wild Salmon | 63 |
| Strips of Chicken Barbecue Wrap | 65 |
| Green Fatty Pizza | 66 |
| Veggies and Cottage Cheese Dip | 68 |
| Fruit and Dark Greens Salad | 69 |
| Grenade Salad | 71 |
| Quinoa-based Asian Salad | 72 |
| Orange-Walnut Salad | 73 |
| Chicken Salad Broccoli with Olive Oil | 74 |
| Cobb and Egg Salad | 75 |
| Asian Stir-Fry | 76 |
| Horseradish Aioli and Roast Beef Sandwich | 77 |
| Kale, Lentils, and Onion Pasta | 78 |
| Barley and Chicken Soup | 80 |
| Chia Seed and Strawberry Pudding | 82 |
| Strawberry Smoothie | 83 |
| Poached Egg Mytilene | 84 |
| Veggie Omelet and Avocado Shake | 85 |
| Bean Soup and Greens | 86 |
| **A 2-Week Plan to Start Managing Adult Scoliosis** | **88** |
| Week 1 | 88 |
| Week 2 | 92 |
| **Conclusion** | **95** |
| Final Thoughts on Managing Adult Scoliosis | 95 |
| **FAQs** | **98** |
| **References and Helpful Links** | **101** |

# Introduction

Adult scoliosis refers to a lateral curvature of the spine that can develop at any stage of life. It affects approximately 6 to 9 million individuals in the United States, accounting for 2-3% of the population. A two-decade-long study found that around 40% of adults with scoliosis experienced varying degrees of bone abnormalities over time.

Although scoliosis is most often identified during adolescence, it can also develop in adulthood. Adult scoliosis may arise from degenerative changes in the spine or as a leftover curve from adolescent scoliosis. Common symptoms include persistent back pain, feelings of fatigue, and, in some cases, difficulty with breathing.

There is no cure for adult scoliosis, but there are treatments that can help ease symptoms and prevent the condition from getting worse.

Diet is an important part of managing adult scoliosis. Certain foods can help to reduce inflammation and pain, and some foods should be avoided. In this guide, you will learn which foods to eat and which to avoid, as well as sample recipes and a two-week meal plan.

In this guide, we will talk about the following:

- What adult scoliosis is
- It's symptoms and risk factors
- How it's diagnosed
- Psychological and Emotional Impact of Scoliosis
- Natural Methods to Manage Adult Scoliosis
- Technological and Medical Advances in Scoliosis Management
- Case Studies and Success Stories
- Support Systems for Scoliosis Patients and Caregivers
- Therapy and exercises for scoliosis
- The right diet for adult scoliosis

Keep reading to learn more about how you can manage your adult scoliosis through proper diet and nutrition. By the end of this guide, you will have a better understanding of how food can impact your condition and discover new ways to improve your overall health.

# What Is Adult Scoliosis?

Adult scoliosis is a sideways curvature of the spine that can occur at any age. While it is most commonly diagnosed in adolescents, it can also affect adults. The word scoliosis comes from the Greek word "skoliose," which means "crooked."

The spine is a column of bone that extends from the base of the skull to the pelvis. It is made up of 33 individual bones, called vertebrae, that are stacked on top of each other. In between each vertebra is a gel-like cushion, called a disc, that acts as a shock absorber for the spine. The spine also contains several ligaments and muscles that help to keep it stable.

The vertebrae are divided into three main sections: the cervical (neck), thoracic (chest), and lumbar (lower back) regions. The bones in each region are numbered according to their location, with the cervical vertebrae being labeled C1 to C7, the thoracic vertebrae T1 to T12, and the lumbar vertebrae L1 to L5. The bones of the spine are connected by a series of joints called facet joints.

The spinal cord is a long, thin bundle of nerves that runs through the center of the spine. It carries messages between the brain and the rest of the body. The spinal cord is protected by the vertebrae, as well as by a layer of tissue called the dura mater.

The nerves that branch off from the spinal cord are arranged in pairs. Each pair consists of one dorsal (back) nerve and one ventral (front) nerve. These nerves exit the spinal cord through small openings between the vertebrae, called foramina.

The spinal column is curved in a gentle S-shape when viewed from the side. This normal curvature helps to absorb shock and distribute weight evenly throughout the spine. When the spine curves excessively to either side, it is called scoliosis.

Scoliosis can occur in any region of the spine, but it most commonly affects the thoracic and/or lumbar regions.

The condition may be classified according to the location of the curve:

- ***Thoracic scoliosis:*** Curvature of the thoracic spine. The most common type of scoliosis is characterized by an S-shaped or C-shaped curvature. This condition is characterized by a curvature of the spine in the thoracic (upper back) region. The spine may have an S-shaped or C-shaped curve. Thoracic means "of the

chest," and this type of scoliosis is named for the location of the curve.
- ***Lumbar scoliosis:*** Curvature of the lumbar spine. The second most common type of scoliosis, lumbar scoliosis is characterized by a curve in the lower back region. The word Lumbar means "of the loin or lower back," and this type of scoliosis is named for the location of the curve.
- ***Cervical scoliosis:*** Curvature of the cervical spine. This is the least common form of scoliosis, and it is characterized by a curve in the neck region. The word Cervical means "of the neck," and this type of scoliosis is named for the location of the curve.
- ***Thoracolumbar scoliosis:*** Curvature of both the thoracic and lumbar spine. This type of scoliosis is a combination of thoracic and lumbar scoliosis, and it is characterized by a curvature in both the upper and lower back regions. The reason for the curvature may be different in each region.
- ***Double major curve scoliosis:*** Curvature of the thoracic and cervical spine, or the lumbar and cervical spine. This type of scoliosis is characterized by a curvature in two regions of the spine (thoracic and cervical).

The severity of scoliosis is determined by the degree of the curve:

- *Mild* – curve measuring 10 to 20 degrees
- *Moderate* – curve measuring 20 to 40 degrees
- *Severe* – curve measuring 40 to 50 degrees
- *Very severe* – curve measuring 50 to 70 degrees

Typically, scoliosis progresses slowly, and the degree of curvature increases as the child grows. In some cases, however, the curve may worsen rapidly. This is more likely to occur in adolescents who are still growing.

## Symptoms

The most common symptom of scoliosis is a noticeable curve in the spine. The degree of curvature will determine the severity of symptoms. In mild cases, there may be no pain or other symptoms. In more severe cases, however, the following symptoms may be present:

- Uneven shoulders
- More prominent shoulder blade compared to the other
- Waist sides are also uneven
- Unbalanced hips
- Looking lopsided
- Pain in the back
- Feeling fatigued

If scoliosis is left untreated, it can lead to several complications, such as:

- **Respiratory problems** – severe scoliosis can interfere with normal breathing by placing pressure on the lungs and heart.
- **Digestive problems** – severe scoliosis can compress the stomach and intestines, making it difficult to digest food properly. It can make you feel full even after eating only a small amount of food.
- **Disability** – in very severe cases, scoliosis can cause disability due to the deformity of the spine.

Early detection and treatment of scoliosis are crucial to prevent complications such as respiratory issues, digestive problems, and disability. If you notice any symptoms, consult a healthcare professional to address the condition promptly.

## Causes

The cause of scoliosis is unknown in most cases. The condition is considered idiopathic, which means that the cause cannot be determined. In some cases, however, scoliosis may be caused by:

- **Congenital scoliosis:** This type of scoliosis is present at birth and is caused by abnormal development of the spine.
- **Neuromuscular scoliosis:** This type of scoliosis is caused by conditions that affect the nervous system and muscles, such as cerebral palsy or muscular dystrophy.

- ***Degenerative scoliosis:*** This type of scoliosis is caused by the breakdown of spinal discs or joints. It is more common in adults over the age of 40.
- ***Idiopathic scoliosis:*** This type of scoliosis has no known cause. The most common form of scoliosis, idiopathic scoliosis can affect anyone at any age, but it is most common in adolescents between the ages of 10 and 15.

Scoliosis can arise from various causes, including congenital, neuromuscular, degenerative, or idiopathic factors. Understanding these types helps in identifying the underlying condition and guiding appropriate treatment.

## Risk Factors for Developing Scoliosis

While scoliosis can affect anyone, certain factors may increase the likelihood of developing the condition. These include:

- ***Family History:*** Genetics can play a role. If you or other family members have scoliosis, your child may have a higher chance of developing it. Monitoring for early signs is particularly important in these cases.
- ***Gender:*** Girls are at a higher risk of scoliosis than boys, especially when it comes to more severe curves that may require treatment.
- ***Age:*** Scoliosis most commonly appears during the rapid growth spurt that occurs just before puberty,

typically between the ages of 10 and 15. Regular checkups during these developmental years can help with early detection.

Understanding and recognizing these risk factors can help ensure early diagnosis and prompt management of scoliosis for better outcomes.

## Prevention

There is currently no known way to prevent scoliosis, as its exact causes are often unclear and can depend on a variety of genetic and environmental factors. However, early detection plays a crucial role in managing the condition. Regular check-ups, especially during childhood and adolescence when scoliosis is most likely to develop, can help identify the condition early.

Early diagnosis allows for timely treatment, which may involve bracing or physical therapy to manage symptoms and potentially prevent the condition from worsening. Proactive monitoring is key to addressing scoliosis effectively.

## Diagnosis

Scoliosis is typically diagnosed during a physical exam. Your doctor will look for signs of a curve in the spine and will measure the degree of curvature with a device called a scoliometer. A scoliometer is a curved ruler that is placed on the back. The degree of curvature is determined by how far the scoliometer deviates from being level.

The *Cobb angle* is the most common method of measuring scoliosis. It is the angle between the uppermost and lowest points of the curve, as seen from the side. The bigger the Cobb angle, the more severe the deformity.

Your doctor may also ask you to perform a *forward bend test*. This involves standing straight with your feet together and your hands on your hips. Your doctor will then ask you to bend forward at the waist. This test is used to assess the severity of the curve and to look for any signs of spinal deformity.

In addition, your doctor may ask you questions about your medical history and family history.

Other methods for assessing scoliosis severity include taking an X-ray. This imaging test can show the degree of curvature and any changes that have occurred over time. This is a type of electromagnetic radiation, which means they are made up of waves of electric and magnetic energy moving through space at the speed of light.

X-rays can penetrate the body, which makes them useful for imaging. They are most commonly used to examine the bones and teeth, but can also be used to look at the lungs, heart, and other organs. X-rays are made by passing a stream of electrons through a metal target. The electrons collide with the atoms in the metal, causing them to emit X-rays.

Different materials absorb X-rays to different degrees. This is what makes it possible to create images of the inside of the body. Bones, for example, absorb more X-rays than soft tissues such as the lungs.

X-rays are detected by special film or digital detectors. The film is placed on the body part being imaged, and the X-rays make a latent image on the film. This image is then developed in a darkroom or viewed digitally.

***CT scan:*** This imaging test can provide a more detailed view of the spine than an X-ray.

***MRI:*** This imaging test can provide a detailed view of the spine and surrounding structures.

Scoliosis is diagnosed through physical exams, imaging tests like X-rays, and assessments such as the Cobb angle and forward bend test to determine the severity of the curve. Advanced imaging methods like CT scans or MRIs may be used for more detailed evaluations when necessary.

## Treatment for Scoliosis

The primary goal of scoliosis treatment is to prevent the curve from worsening and to manage pain. The best treatment depends on the severity of the condition and individual factors. Here's an overview of common options:

- ***Observation:*** For mild scoliosis, observation is typically recommended. This involves regular check-ups to monitor the curve's progression. If the curve remains stable, no further intervention may be necessary.
- ***Bracing:*** Bracing is often prescribed for moderate scoliosis to prevent the curve from worsening. A spinal brace, made from plastic, metal, or a combination of materials, is designed to fit snugly around the torso. It supports the spine and stabilizes the curve. Adjustable and secured with Velcro or buckles, braces allow for a customized fit based on individual needs. Consistent use, as advised by your doctor, can be key in slowing progression.
- ***Surgery:*** Surgery may be recommended for severe scoliosis, especially when the curve is causing significant pain or affecting quality of life. The most common procedure is spinal fusion, using metal rods, screws, or other devices to correct and stabilize the spine. Surgery can help prevent further deterioration and relieve discomfort in advanced cases.

Each treatment aims to restore spinal stability and improve overall function. Work closely with your healthcare provider to find the option that best suits your needs and to ensure your condition is effectively managed.

# Psychological and Emotional Impact of Scoliosis

Living with scoliosis is more than just managing a curved spine; it entails navigating a range of psychological and emotional challenges that can significantly affect quality of life. For many individuals, scoliosis doesn't just affect the body—it impacts self-esteem, mental health, and overall well-being. Understanding these challenges, while exploring ways to cope, can empower those living with scoliosis to feel supported and in control.

## Mental Health Challenges Faced by Scoliosis Patients

Dealing with scoliosis can trigger a myriad of negative emotions, including anxiety, depression, and social isolation. It's normal for individuals to feel overwhelmed by the diagnosis and the demands of treatment, especially if surgery is required.

The physical changes brought on by scoliosis may also cause self-esteem issues and feelings of body image dissatisfaction.

These emotional struggles can be exacerbated during adolescence, as appearance often plays a significant role in self-identity and peer relationships.

1. **Anxiety About Appearance**

    The visible effects of scoliosis can make some individuals feel self-conscious about their appearance. Curvature of the spine, uneven shoulders, or hips often draw unwanted attention or comments, which can fuel anxiety in social situations. Adolescents, in particular, may feel immense pressure to fit societal standards of beauty, making it hard to accept their body as it is.

2. **Self-Esteem and Body Image Issues**

    Anxiety about appearance can easily tie into more complex struggles with self-esteem and body image. Feeling "different" or misunderstood because of scoliosis may lead to feelings of isolation. This emotional toll isn't restricted to a specific age group—anyone living with scoliosis can experience this at some point, especially during times of change or stress.

3. **The Emotional Toll of Chronic Pain**

    Chronic pain is a reality for many scoliosis patients, and it can take a significant toll on emotional well-being. Living with persistent discomfort can lead to frustration, irritability, or even depressive symptoms.

It's overwhelming to face pain that interferes with daily activities, sleep, or one's ability to fully enjoy life. Over time, unaddressed pain can blur the line between physical and emotional challenges, creating a cycle that's hard to break.

## Strategies for Emotional Well-Being

While scoliosis presents unique emotional hurdles, there are ways to cultivate resilience and emotional balance. Simple, intentional steps can provide both short-term relief and long-term empowerment.

1. **Practice Mindfulness**

   Mindfulness is a powerful tool for managing anxiety and stress. Techniques like deep breathing, meditation, or body scanning can help you reconnect with the present moment instead of being consumed by worries about your pain or appearance. Apps, online videos, or local workshops can serve as a great introduction to mindfulness if you're new to it.

2. **Connect With Support Groups**

   Sometimes, the most comforting thing is knowing you're not alone. Support groups—whether online or in person—can connect you with others who truly understand the challenges of living with scoliosis.

These connections foster a sense of belonging, offer valuable advice, and can transform how you view your experience. A strong community can ease feelings of isolation and provide encouragement when you need it most.

3. **Seek Therapy or Counseling**

    Therapy can be a proactive way to address the mental health impacts of scoliosis. A therapist can help you unpack complex emotions, improve self-esteem, or develop coping mechanisms for managing pain and stress. Cognitive-behavioral therapy (CBT) in particular is effective for reframing negative thinking patterns and building confidence. Therapy isn't a sign of weakness—it's an investment in your well-being.

4. **Build a Strong Support Network**

    Your loved ones—whether friends or family—can be a vital part of your emotional healing. Share your struggles with those you trust, and don't hesitate to ask for help when you need it. Even something as simple as venting your frustrations or asking for a hand with daily tasks can lighten the emotional load. Together, your network can remind you that you're supported and valued.

### 5. Keep Moving Forward With Gentle Exercise

Though it may feel counterintuitive, movement can actually benefit both your body and mind. Engaging in activities like yoga, swimming, or gentle stretches can relieve tension caused by scoliosis while also boosting your mood. Movement releases endorphins, the body's natural "feel-good" chemicals, which can help you feel more balanced emotionally.

Scoliosis may bring challenges, but it doesn't define you. Whether dealing with pain, anxiety, or mental health struggles, your experiences are valid, and you're not alone. With tools like mindfulness, therapy, and support, you can build confidence and resilience. You are more than your condition and deserve care and compassion, especially from yourself.

# Natural Methods to Manage Adult Scoliosis

If you are living with adult scoliosis, you can use some natural methods to manage your condition. These include:

## Exercise

Another way to manage adult scoliosis is through exercise. Exercise is important for overall health and well-being. It is also important for maintaining bone health and muscle strength.

Exercise can also help to relieve pain and improve your range of motion. When exercising, it is essential to focus on exercises that strengthen the back and abdominal muscles. These muscles support the spine and help to prevent further curvature.

*Swimming and yoga* are two good examples of exercises that can help to strengthen the back and abdominal muscles.

*Yoga* is a wonderful way to help alleviate the pain and discomfort of adult scoliosis. It is important to find a class specifically geared towards beginners with scoliosis, as some poses may exacerbate your condition. Once you have found a class that feels comfortable for you, there are a few things to keep in mind to get the most out of your practice.

1. ***Listen to your body.*** This is especially important in yoga, as you are working with your breath and body to move in ways that may be unfamiliar. If a pose feels uncomfortable or aggravates your pain, please listen to your body and come out of the pose.
2. ***Talk to your teacher.*** Let them know about your scoliosis so that they can give you modifications or help you find alternative poses that will be more beneficial for you.
3. ***Breathe.*** This may seem like a no-brainer, but it is especially important in yoga to focus on your breath. Taking deep, even breaths will help you to relax and focus on the present moment.
4. ***Have patience.*** Remember that you are just starting out, and it takes time to build strength and flexibility. Don't get discouraged if you can't do a pose perfectly or can only hold it for a short period. Just keep practicing and your body will eventually catch up.
5. ***Have fun!*** Yoga is meant to be a relaxing and enjoyable experience, so make sure to find a class that you enjoy and make the most of it!

# Chiropractic Care

Chiropractic care is another option for managing adult scoliosis. Chiropractors are trained to diagnose and treat conditions of the musculoskeletal system. They use a variety of techniques, such as spinal manipulation, to realign the spine and improve function. Chiropractic care may help to relieve pain, improve range of motion, and prevent further curvature of the spine.

If you think you may have scoliosis, it is important to seek out professional help. A chiropractor can help diagnose scoliosis and develop a treatment plan. When looking for a chiropractor, it is crucial to find one who is experienced in treating scoliosis. You can ask your regular doctor for a referral, or you can search for a chiropractor online. Once you have found a few potential chiropractors, you should call and ask about their experience in treating scoliosis. You should also ask about the treatment methods they use.

**What to expect from your first visit**

During your first visit, the chiropractor will likely take a medical history and ask about your symptoms. They will then do a physical exam. This may include checking your posture and examining your spine. The chiropractor may also order X-rays or other imaging tests to get a better look at your spine. Once the chiropractor has all of the information they need, they will develop a treatment plan.

## Massage Therapy

Massage therapy is another option for managing adult scoliosis. Massage therapists use a variety of techniques to relax the muscles and relieve pain. Massage therapy may help to improve range of motion, reduce muscle tension, and relieve pain.

When looking for a massage therapist, again, find someone who is experienced in treating scoliosis. Also, referrals from your doctor are great because you can rely on their professionalism. Make sure that you do more research and, if possible, interview the therapist to ask them about their experience and the types of massages they do to treat scoliosis.

Additionally, there's also the Schroth Method, which is a physical therapy approach to treating scoliosis. Mainly, its treatment, or exercise, is tailored to the type of curvature the spine has. Because this is a customized form of treatment, it's important to consult with an expert if you're interested in trying out this program. Make sure that you also consult with your doctor prior to trying out the Schroth program.

### What to expect from your first visit

During your first visit, the massage therapist will likely take a medical history and ask about your symptoms. They will then do a physical exam. This may include checking your posture and examining your spine. The massage therapist will then choose the type of massage they think will be most helpful for you.

## Acupuncture

Acupuncture is another option for managing adult scoliosis. It's a traditional medicine all the way from China. It is done by piercing the skin on specific body parts called points with thin needles. Acupuncture is thought to improve overall health and well-being by restoring balance within the body. It is also believed to relieve pain, improve range of motion, and reduce muscle tension. Studies have shown that acupuncture may have a positive effect on scoliosis.

When looking for an acupuncturist, it is important to find one who is experienced in treating scoliosis. You can ask your regular doctor for a referral, or you can search for an acupuncturist online. Once you have found a few potential acupuncturists, you should call and ask about their experience in treating scoliosis.

### What to expect from your first visit

During your first visit, the acupuncturist will likely take a medical history and ask about your symptoms. They will then choose the points on your body that they will need to insert the needles into. The needles are usually inserted into the skin at a depth of zero.

# Herbal Medicine

Herbal medicine is another option for managing adult scoliosis. Herbal medicine is the use of plants to treat medical conditions. Herbal medicines are thought to be safe and effective for many people. They are often used in combination with other forms of treatment, such as exercise and acupuncture. Herbal medicines that are thought to be beneficial for scoliosis include ginger and turmeric.

These herbs are anti-inflammatory and help to reduce pain and muscle tension. Herbal medicines are available in many forms, such as capsules, tinctures, and teas.

When looking for an herbalist, find one who is experienced in treating scoliosis. You can ask your regular doctor for a referral, or you can search for an herbalist online. Once you have found a few potential herbalists, you should call and ask about their experience in treating scoliosis. You should also ask about the type of herbal medicine they use.

## What to expect from your first visit

During your first visit, the herbalist will likely take a medical history and ask about your symptoms. They will then choose the herbs that they think will be most helpful for you. Herbal medicines are available in many forms, such as capsules, tinctures, and teas.

# Daily Living with Scoliosis

Living with scoliosis can come with its challenges, but there are ways to make daily life more comfortable and manageable. Simple adjustments to how you sit, sleep, and move, along with the right tools, can help you ease discomfort and protect your back. Below are some practical tips to support you in your daily routine with scoliosis.

## Ergonomics Tips for Scoliosis

1. **Posture Matters**

   Sitting for long periods can be tough on your back, especially with scoliosis. Maintaining good posture is key to reducing strain. Here are a few tips for sitting comfortably:

   - Sit with your back straight and both feet flat on the floor.
   - Avoid slouching or leaning to one side, as this can put extra pressure on the curve in your spine.

- Choose a chair with good lumbar support, or add a small cushion behind your lower back for extra comfort.
- Take regular breaks to stand up, stretch, and move around to prevent stiffness.

2. **Sleeping Positions**

The way you sleep can also affect how your back feels when you wake up. A good sleeping posture can help align your spine and minimize discomfort. Try these tips for better rest:

- Sleep on your back with a supportive pillow under your knees to reduce pressure on your lower spine.
- If you prefer sleeping on your side, use a body pillow or place a cushion between your knees. This helps keep your hips and spine aligned.
- Avoid sleeping on your stomach, as it can strain your back and neck.

## Helpful Daily Aids

The right tools can make your day-to-day life a lot easier when you have scoliosis. Below are some recommendations for products that offer extra support and comfort.

1. **Supportive Pillows**

   Investing in quality pillows can make a huge difference, whether you're sitting or sleeping.

   - Lumbar Support Cushions: Ideal for use at work, in the car, or at home, these pillows help maintain proper back alignment.
   - Contour Pillows: These are great for aligning your neck and spine while you sleep, reducing tension and discomfort.

2. **Back Braces**

   A back brace can provide additional support and help you maintain better posture throughout the day.

   - Talk to your doctor or a specialist to find one that's suited to your specific needs. A properly fitted brace can help reduce pain and pressure on your spine.
   - Make sure to follow usage instructions carefully, as wearing a brace too often or incorrectly can cause more harm than good.

3. **Ergonomic Accessories**

   Small ergonomic adjustments can go a long way in making everyday tasks easier.

   - Use an adjustable standing desk if you spend long hours working at a computer. This

encourages better posture by allowing you to alternate between sitting and standing.
- Look for backpacks with padded straps and multiple compartments to evenly distribute weight, especially if you carry heavy items often.

Managing scoliosis is about finding what works best for you and your body. Paying close attention to ergonomics, investing in helpful tools, and making small adjustments to your daily habits can lead to big improvements in your comfort and overall quality of life.

And remember, you don't have to figure it all out on your own. Consulting with a physical therapist, doctor, or other experts can help you discover even more ways to stay comfortable and protect your back.

## Scoliosis-Specific Exercise Programs

Exercise plays a vital role in managing scoliosis and improving quality of life. It can help strengthen the core, increase flexibility, and support better posture, all of which are essential for reducing pain and improving spinal alignment.

Doing the right exercises consistently can empower you to take an active role in managing your condition. Below is a comprehensive guide to scoliosis-specific exercises, along with tips on how to perform them safely and effectively.

**Core-Strengthening Exercises**

A strong core stabilizes the spine and reduces stress on the muscles and joints, crucial for individuals dealing with scoliosis. Core exercises also promote balance, helping to correct uneven posture.

1. **Plank Variations**
   - *Standard Plank:* Start in a prone position, supporting your weight on your forearms and toes. Keep your body in a straight line from head to heels. Tighten your core and hold the position for 20-60 seconds.
   - *Knee Plank (Modified):* Perform the plank on your knees to reduce strain if you're just starting. Progress to a full plank as you build strength.
   - *Side Plank:* Lie on one side, balancing on one forearm and the side of your foot. Keep your body straight and hold for 15-30 seconds on each side. This targets oblique muscles that are essential for spinal stability.
2. **Bird-Dog**
   - Start on your hands and knees in a tabletop position.

- Extend one arm straight out in front and the opposite leg straight behind you, forming a straight line from hand to foot.
- Hold for 5 seconds, focusing on keeping your core tight, then return to the starting position and switch sides.

3. **Dead Bug**
    - Lie on your back with your arms extended toward the ceiling and knees bent at 90 degrees.
    - Lower one arm and the opposite leg until they're just above the floor, then return to the starting position and repeat with the other side.

These exercises focus on improving strength and stability in the lumbar and thoracic regions, which often bear the brunt of scoliosis-related strain.

**Flexibility and Range of Motion**

Improving flexibility can ease muscle tension and help the body adapt to spinal asymmetry. Incorporate these stretches into your routine for better mobility:

1. **Cat-Cow Stretch**
    - Start in a tabletop position on your hands and knees.
    - Arch your back upwards into a "cat" stretch, tucking your chin toward your chest.

- Reverse the position, lowering your belly and lifting your head and tailbone ("cow" stretch).
- Perform the movement 10 to 15 times at a gentle pace, concentrating on improving spinal mobility.

2. **Child's Pose with Side Stretch**
   - Kneel on the floor and sit back on your heels.
   - Extend your arms forward, placing your palms on the floor, and lower your chest towards the ground.
   - To stretch a specific side, walk your hands to either side, feeling a gentle pull along the spine and side body. Hold each side for 30 seconds.

3. **Seated Spinal Twist**
   - Sit with both legs extended in front of you.
   - Bend one knee and cross it over the opposite extended leg.
   - Place the opposite arm behind your bent knee and twist your torso gently toward the bent leg.
   - Hold for 20-30 seconds, then switch sides.

Flexibility exercises are gentle yet effective at releasing tension in tight areas like the hips, lower back, and shoulders—key regions affected by scoliosis.

**Posture Correction Routines**

Correcting posture is a central part of managing scoliosis. These exercises aim to realign the spine, strengthen postural muscles, and prevent further curvatures.

1. **Wall Angels**
    - Stand with your back against a wall, feet a few inches away, and lower back gently pressed into the wall.
    - Raise your arms to form a "goalpost" position, with elbows bent at 90 degrees.
    - Slowly move your arms upward, as if making a snow angel, then lower them back down. Aim for 10 repetitions while keeping your back in contact with the wall throughout.
2. **Reverse Fly with Resistance Band**
    - Hold a resistance band in both hands, arms straight out in front of you.
    - Stretch the band by bringing your shoulder blades together while maintaining straight arms.
    - Return to the starting position and repeat for 15 repetitions.
3. **Scapular Retractions**
    - Keep your back straight while sitting or standing.
    - Bring your shoulder blades together as if you're pinching a pencil between them.

- Hold the position for 5 seconds, then release. Repeat 10-15 times.

4. **Cobra Stretch**
    - Lie face down on the floor with your hands placed under your shoulders.
    - Gently push your upper body upward, lifting your chest off the ground while keeping your pelvis in contact with the floor.
    - Hold for 15-20 seconds and release, repeating 5 times.

Posture-correction exercises train the upper back, shoulders, and neck to maintain proper alignment, reducing compensatory imbalances.

**Videos and Visual Aids**

- *YouTube Channels:* Look for channels like "Yoga with Adriene" (for scoliosis-friendly yoga) or "Bob & Brad" (physical therapy exercises).
- *Schroth Method Videos:* Search for "Schroth Method scoliosis exercises" on YouTube for demonstrations tailored to scoliosis.
- *Pilates for Scoliosis:* Channels like "Pilatesology" often provide scoliosis-specific routines.

**Safety Tips When Exercising with Scoliosis**

- *Consult Your Doctor:* Before starting any new exercise routine, confirm which movements are safe for your specific curvature and degree of scoliosis.
- *Listen to Your Body:* Avoid exercises that cause sharp pain or discomfort. Soreness is normal, but pain may indicate improper form or strain.
- *Use Mirrors:* When possible, exercise in front of a mirror to check your alignment and ensure proper form.
- *Go Slow:* Focus on controlled movements. Rapid or jerky actions can exacerbate discomfort and irritation in the spine.
- *Warm-Up and Cool Down:* Always prepare your muscles and joints with easy stretches before progressing to core or strength exercises.

Consistency is key to reaping the benefits of these exercises. Begin with two or three sessions per week, gradually increasing intensity as your strength and comfort improve. Remember, every small effort contributes to a healthier and more supportive spine.

By incorporating these scoliosis-specific exercises into your life, you're building a foundation for better posture, greater flexibility, and reduced discomfort.

# Technological and Medical Advances in Scoliosis Management

Modern medicine has made immense strides in the diagnosis and treatment of scoliosis, providing both patients and healthcare providers with innovative tools and techniques to improve outcomes. Technological and medical advancements now make it possible to manage scoliosis more effectively, with less pain and disruption to a patient's lifestyle.

Here, we'll explore some of the latest breakthroughs, from cutting-edge diagnostic tools to next-generation treatments that are reshaping scoliosis care.

## Advancements in Non-Invasive Diagnostics

Non-invasive diagnostic tools are revolutionizing scoliosis management by providing faster, more accurate spinal assessments while reducing the need for frequent X-rays, making them ideal for long-term monitoring.

1. ***Surface Topography Systems:*** Surface topography uses light-based technology to create a three-dimensional map of the spine's surface without

the need for radiation. Devices like the Scoliometer and Moiré Topography scan the contour of the back and identify asymmetries indicative of scoliosis. These tools are painless, non-invasive, and provide instant feedback, making them ideal for regular monitoring of mild to moderate curvatures.

2. *EOS Imaging System:* This state-of-the-art imaging system delivers detailed 3D models of the spine, hips, and lower limbs using ultra-low-dose radiation. Unlike traditional X-rays, EOS imaging allows doctors to view a full-body scan in weight-bearing positions, offering a more comprehensive understanding of spinal alignment and its effects on surrounding structures.

3. *AI-Assisted Diagnosis:* Artificial Intelligence (AI) is now used to analyze imaging results with exceptional precision. Machine learning algorithms can measure curvature angles, classify scoliosis types, and even predict the likelihood of future progression based on specific spinal data. This helps doctors recommend tailored treatment strategies.

These advancements in non-invasive diagnostics are transforming scoliosis management by providing safer, faster, and more precise assessments. With tools like surface topography, EOS imaging, and AI-powered analysis, patients can benefit from improved monitoring and personalized treatment strategies.

# Minimally Invasive Treatments

For patients requiring treatment beyond observation, minimally invasive options are reshaping how scoliosis is managed—and with significantly reduced risks and recovery time compared to traditional surgical methods.

1. *Minimally Invasive Spinal Fusion Surgery:* Traditional spinal fusion surgery involves creating large incisions along the back, which can lead to significant post-operative pain and extended recovery periods. Today, minimally invasive approaches use advanced navigation systems and smaller incisions to stabilize spinal curvature while minimizing damage to surrounding tissues. These techniques significantly reduce recovery times, allowing patients to return to normal activities faster.
2. *Vertebral Body Tethering (VBT):* Vertebral body tethering is a groundbreaking surgical technique that uses flexible cords instead of rigid metal rods to address abnormal spinal curves. The tether is attached to screws placed on individual vertebrae and tightened to correct curvature. Unlike traditional methods, VBT allows for continued growth and flexibility, making it a popular choice for younger patients or individuals with mild-to-moderate scoliosis.
3. *Injection-Based Pain Management:* For adults with scoliosis-related chronic pain, minimally invasive

injection therapies like epidural steroid injections or nerve blocks can target inflammation and provide temporary relief. These procedures are quick, effective, and often used in conjunction with physical therapy.

Minimally invasive treatments are transforming scoliosis care by offering effective solutions with reduced risks and faster recovery times. From advanced surgeries like VBT to pain management injections, these approaches provide patients with safer, more flexible options tailored to their needs.

## Emerging Therapies and Technologies

The future of scoliosis management is incredibly promising, with new and emerging therapies that push the boundaries of what is possible. These innovations are designed to make treatments more personalized, accurate, and patient-friendly.

1. ***Robotic-Assisted Surgery:*** Robotic systems, such as the Mazor X or ROSA Spine platforms, are revolutionizing scoliosis surgery by increasing precision and safety. These systems provide surgeons with a virtual blueprint of the spine, allowing for highly accurate placement of screws and rods. The use of robotics reduces intraoperative risks and shortens recovery time for patients.
2. ***3D-Printed Braces:*** Traditional back braces can be uncomfortable and aesthetically unappealing, often

making compliance difficult for patients. Enter 3D-printed braces, which are custom-designed using advanced imaging tools to ensure a perfect fit. These braces are lightweight, discreet, and highly effective. They not only improve patient comfort but also enhance treatment results by providing targeted pressure on specific areas of the spine.
3. *Exoskeleton-Assisted Therapy:* Exoskeletons—a form of wearable robotics—are being explored as therapy tools to improve spinal alignment, mobility, and muscle engagement. These devices offer personalized movement support, which can potentially reduce pain and improve posture over time.
4. *Tissue Engineering and Biomaterials:* Innovators in the field of regenerative medicine are investigating the use of stem cells and biologically engineered materials to repair or replace damaged spinal discs. Preliminary research suggests that these techniques could one day provide a non-surgical solution to degenerative scoliosis.
5. *Enhanced Scoliosis Monitoring with Wearable Devices:* Smart wearable devices, such as posture-correcting gadgets and scoliosis-specific trackers, are enabling patients to monitor their spinal alignment and mobility in real time. These devices alert the wearer to poor posture or other habits that

could exacerbate spinal curves, integrating scoliosis management seamlessly into daily life.

Advancements in scoliosis care are transforming treatment with precision and patient-focused solutions. Non-invasive diagnostics enable early detection, while minimally invasive treatments and innovations like robotic-assisted surgeries and 3D-printed braces offer faster recovery and better outcomes. Speak to a healthcare professional to explore these cutting-edge options for improved spinal health.

# Case Studies and Success Stories

**Josie**

Josie's story highlights the incredible impact of non-surgical scoliosis treatment. Starting her care at 10 years old, Josie saw her Cobb angle improve significantly, from 37° to under 9°. Over five years, her hard work paid off, allowing her to live free from the side effects of surgery.

Josie's family celebrated her progress, and she has since pursued her dreams of modeling and continued playing volleyball. Reflecting on her experience, Josie shared, "It was well worth the hard work." Her success shows how a personalized, non-invasive approach can lead to lasting results and a fulfilling, active lifestyle.

**Randy**

Randy, an adult scoliosis patient, struggled with growing back pain over the years. He tried managing it with treatments like physical therapy and pain medication but found no lasting results. Eventually, in his 50s, he opted for scoliosis surgery performed by Dr. Richard Hostin. The procedure involved rods and screws from T5 to his pelvis.

Randy shared how the surgery changed his life, allowing him to enjoy his daily activities again. Dr. Hostin explained, "We measure our success by our patients' expectations of success." Thanks to this care, Randy now lives pain-free and with renewed joy in his life.

**Marcia**

Marcia's scoliosis surgery changed her life for the better. After years of pain and limited mobility, her curve had progressed to 70 degrees, making basic tasks like walking incredibly difficult. Post-surgery, she worked hard to regain strength and celebrated milestones, like walking up her steep driveway and swimming again.

She shared, "My first big 'Aha' moment came when I walked around the Denver Zoo with my grandson for 2½ hours with no back pain." Later, she returned to skiing, a lifelong dream, and felt like her true self again. Marcia's story shows the incredible possibilities after choosing expert care.

**Lorri**

"At the time, I felt like I was stuck in my crooked body for life and all hope was lost." Despite challenges, including teasing, job limitations, and personal hardships, Lorri never gave up. Through consistent chiropractic care, she saw improvements in her posture and muscle strain, giving her a sense of relief and hope.

Lorri's journey highlights her strength and determination to keep fighting, even when life felt overwhelming. Her story inspires others to explore non-surgical options and believe in the possibility of a better future.

## Support Systems for Scoliosis Patients and Caregivers

Managing scoliosis can be challenging for both patients and their caregivers, but there are numerous support systems available to provide assistance, encouragement, and guidance. Below is a detailed list of resources to help you find the support you need.

### Online Support Groups

1. *Scoliosis Support on Inspire.com:* A community forum where patients and caregivers can discuss their experiences, share advice, and find encouragement from others dealing with scoliosis. The platform offers groups for specific topics like bracing, surgery, and pain management.
2. *Curvy Girls Scoliosis Foundation:* This global network connects young girls with scoliosis, creating a space where they can share their journeys. They offer online meetups, educational resources, and tips to boost confidence during treatment.
3. *Scoliosis Warriors (Facebook Group):* A Facebook community offering a friendly environment for

scoliosis patients of all ages. Participants share their stories, treatment experiences, and tips for coping with daily challenges.
4. ***ScoliSMART Forum:*** A platform focused on non-surgical scoliosis treatment solutions, offering advice and support for parents and individuals seeking alternative therapies.
5. ***Reddit's r/Scoliosis Community:*** A subreddit where scoliosis patients can ask questions, swap stories, and discuss all aspects of care in an open and inclusive environment.

**Local Support Groups**

1. ***Scoliosis Association Chapters:*** Local chapters of the National Scoliosis Foundation often host in-person events, workshops, and informational sessions for patients and families. Visit their website to find a chapter near you.
2. ***Hospital-Run Scoliosis Support Groups:*** Many hospitals and orthopedic clinics host scoliosis education and support groups. These sessions allow patients to connect locally while learning about treatment options and coping strategies.
3. ***YMCA or Community Centers:*** Some local YMCA programs or community centers host scoliosis-specific fitness classes or support groups. These aim to

promote physical well-being and provide a welcoming environment.

**Finding Specialists**
1. *Orthopedic Clinics or Scoliosis Centers:* Start by contacting nearby hospitals or scoliosis-specific treatment centers like the CLEAR Institute or Scoliosis Reduction Center. These locations often have experts including chiropractors, physical therapists, and scoliosis-focused care teams.
2. *Scoliosis Therapists:* Use directories like the American Physical Therapy Association (APTA) or CLEAR Institute to find therapists certified in scoliosis-specific methods such as the Schroth method or CLEAR principles.
3. *Dietitians:* Platforms like the Academy of Nutrition and Dietetics can help identify dietitians specializing in musculoskeletal health. A healthy diet can support bone health and improve overall recovery and well-being.
4. *Chiropractors:* Reach out to licensed chiropractors through directories like the International Chiropractic Pediatric Association (ICPA). Look for those with experience in scoliosis-focused chiropractic care.

## Helpful Tips for Finding Support

- *Ask for References:* Ask your primary care physician or orthopedic surgeon for recommendations when searching for specialists or local support groups.
- *Research Local Nonprofits:* Organizations like the Scoliosis Research Society or Scoliosis Association often list local resources and contacts.
- *Join Webinars and Events:* Many scoliosis-focused organizations host online webinars and treatment Q&A sessions, providing direct connections to knowledgeable professionals.

By combining these online and in-person resources with support from caregivers and specialists, scoliosis patients can access the guidance and encouragement needed to manage their condition effectively.

# Managing Adult Scoliosis Through Diet

One of the ways you can manage adult scoliosis is through diet. Eating a healthy, balanced diet is vital for overall health and well-being. It is also important for maintaining bone health.

## List of Foods to Consume

If you have adult scoliosis, there are certain foods you should eat more of to help manage your condition.

Among these are foods high in calcium and vitamin D, such as:

- Yogurt
- Cheese
- Milk
- Canned fish with bones (such as salmon and sardines)
- Dark leafy greens (such as kale and spinach)
- Broccoli
- Oranges
- Beans

- Peas
- Wild-caught salmon
- Pasture-raised Eggs

***Calcium*** is the most abundant mineral in the human body, making up about 2% of our total body weight. While most of our calcium is stored in our bones and teeth, it's also found in our blood and plays an important role in many of our body's essential functions.

We need calcium for strong bones and teeth, normal blood clotting, proper muscle function, and nervous system function. Our bodies need calcium to build and maintain strong bones. Calcium is also important for proper muscle function and helps our nerves transmit messages throughout our body.

When our bodies don't get enough calcium, we can develop health problems like osteoporosis (a condition that causes bones to become thin and weak) or rickets (a condition that affects bone development in children). Adult scoliosis can also lead to a decrease in bone density, which makes calcium even more important for people with the condition.

***Vitamin D*** is a fat-soluble vitamin that our bodies need for calcium absorption, bone health, and immune function. Vitamin D is found in salmon and tuna, which are considered fatty fish, mushrooms, and egg yolks. However, most of the vitamin D in our bodies comes from exposure to sunlight.

When our bodies are exposed to sunlight, our skin produces vitamin D. This vitamin D is then transported to our liver and kidneys, where it's converted into the active form of vitamin D that our bodies need.

Vitamin D is important for calcium absorption and bone health. It helps our bodies absorb calcium from the food we eat and maintain proper blood levels of calcium. Vitamin D also helps regulate phosphorus levels in our blood and promotes bone growth and remodeling.

You should also eat more fresh fruits and vegetables. Here is a sample list of some of the best ones to eat:

- Strawberries
- Blueberries
- Raspberries
- Blackberries
- Cranberries
- Red peppers
- Green peppers
- Carrots
- Sweet potatoes
- Spinach
- Broccoli
- Kale

However, do limit certain citrus fruits as the acidity can irritate the skin around scoliosis curves. These include oranges, lemons, tomatoes, and limes.

Finally don't shy away from healthy fats. Fats are an important part of a healthy diet and provide essential nutrients.

- Nuts
- Seeds
- Avocados
- Olive oil
- Coconut oil
- Grass-fed butter
- Ghee
- Flaxseed oil
- Fish oil
- Chia

## List of Foods to Avoid

There are some foods that you should avoid if you have scoliosis. These include:

- *Alcohol:* Alcohol can increase the risk of bone loss and may make scoliosis worse.
- *Carbonated Beverages:* carbonated beverages can cause bloating, which may make scoliosis worse.

- ***Caffeine:*** Caffeine can cause dehydration, which can make scoliosis worse.
- ***Salty Foods:*** Salt can cause dehydration, which can make scoliosis worse.
- ***White Flour:*** White flour can cause bloating, which may make scoliosis worse.
- ***Fried Foods:*** Fried foods can cause inflammation, which can make scoliosis worse.
- ***Vegetable Oils:*** Vegetable oils are high in omega-6 fatty acids, which can promote inflammation.
- ***Sugar:*** Sugar can cause weight gain, which may make scoliosis worse.

Finally, avoid processed foods, which is an umbrella term for foods that have been chemically altered or contain artificial ingredients. These foods are often high in sugar, salt, and fat, and can cause weight gain, which may make scoliosis worse.

Processed foods are basically any food that has been altered in some way during manufacturing.

This includes but is not limited to:

- Bread
- Cereal
- Snack foods
- Chips
- Desserts
- Processed meats

- Soda
- Canned fruits and vegetables
- Frozen meals

Processed foods are made using a variety of methods, including canning, freezing, and drying. Some processed foods are also treated with chemicals or other agents to improve their flavor, texture, or shelf life.

While some processed foods can be part of a healthy diet, it's important to limit your intake of these foods and make sure you're eating mostly whole, unprocessed foods.

# Weekly Meal Plan

Ideally, making meal plans is a great way to help you transition from your regular meals to more diet-appropriate choices. Below is a sample meal plan made for a week that you can either follow or modify. The meals used below are based on the sample recipes provided in this guide.

Table 1: Weekly Meal Plan

|       | **Breakfast** | **Lunch** | **Dinner** |
|-------|---------------|-----------|------------|
| Day 1 | Cobb and Egg Salad | Fruit and Dark Greens Salad | Salmon Wrapped in Bacon |
| Day 2 | Barley and Chicken Soup | Veggies and Cottage Cheese Dip | Baked Wild Salmon |
| Day 3 | Grenade Salad | Chicken Salad Broccoli with Olive Oil | Green Fatty Pizza |
| Day 4 | Baked Wild Salmon | Quinoa-based Asian Salad | Barley and Chicken Soup |
| Day 5 | Fruit and Dark Greens Salad | Asian Stir-Fry | Horseradish Aioli and Roast Beef Sandwich |

| Day 6 | Veggies and Cottage Cheese Dip | Strips of Chicken Barbecue Wrap | Kale, Lentils, and Onion Pasta |
|---|---|---|---|
| Day 7 | Chicken Salad Broccoli with Olive Oil | Green Fatty Pizza | Orange-Walnut Salad |

# Sample Recipes

We have included a few sample recipes to help you get started with your weekly meal plan. These recipes are easy to prepare, healthy, and delicious.

# Salmon Wrapped in Bacon

**Ingredients:**

- 2 pcs. 340 g salmon filets, frozen or fresh
- 4 bacon slices
- 1 tbsp. olive oil
- 2 tbsp. tarragon, to garnish
- lemon wedges, to serve

**Instructions:**

1. Preheat the oven to 350°F.
2. Pat dry the salmon filets. Wrap the bacon around each salmon.
3. On a roasting tray, arrange the bacon-wrapped salmon. Use olive oil to drizzle. Bake for 15 to 20 minutes.
4. Garnish with lemon wedges and tarragon. Serve.

# Baked Wild Salmon

**Ingredients:**

- 1.5 lbs. wild salmon
- 2 tbsp. olive oil
- 3 cloves garlic, minced
- 1 tsp. dried oregano
- sea salt
- pepper
- 1 bunch fresh asparagus
- 1/2 cup cucumber
- 1/2 cup tomato, diced
- 1/2 cup feta cheese
- 1/2 cup olives
- 1 whole lemon

**Instructions:**

1. Preheat the oven to 400°F.
2. Line a baking sheet with parchment paper and set aside.
3. Using a small glass bowl, mix oil, oregano, salt, garlic, and pepper. Pour seasoning mix over the salmon and coat the entire fish.
4. Layer the salmon on the baking sheet.
5. Place trimmed asparagus on the sheet pan next to the salmon.

6. Squeeze fresh lemon juice and place the remaining lemon slices on the sheet pan. Bake for 20 minutes.
7. When the salmon is done, serve with a scoop of olive and feta salad over the salmon or on the side, and enjoy.

# Strips of Chicken Barbecue Wrap

**Ingredients:**

- 5 oz. left-over or pre-cooked chicken, cut into strips
- 2 tbsp barbecue sauce
- 1 large whole-grain tortilla
- 1/4 cup broccoli, shredded and blanched
- 1/4 cup carrot, shredded and blanched
- 1/4 cup cauliflower, shredded and blanched
- 1/4 cup cabbage, shredded and blanched

**Instructions:**

1. Put all the shredded vegetables in a bowl and toss to combine well.
2. Spread the tortilla. Put the barbecue sauce, strips of chicken and mixed veggies.
3. Wrap everything, cut in half (secure each half with a toothpick), and serve.

# Green Fatty Pizza

**Ingredients:**

For pizza base:

- 1 whole egg
- 1/2 tsp. dried rosemary
- 2 tbsp. cream cheese
- 85g almond meal
- 170g mozzarella, shredded
- 100g fresh spinach, chopped
- salt, to taste
- pepper, to taste

For pizza toppings:

- 1 medium zucchini, sliced finely
- feta, crumbled
- 1/8 cup spring onion, chopped coarsely
- 1/4 cup fresh mint, chopped coarsely

**Instructions:**

1. Get a microwavable bowl. Put almond flour and mozzarella in it and combine well. Add the cream cheese in.
2. Set the microwave to high and melt the cheese for one minute.
3. Stir the mixture and microwave for another 25 seconds.

4. Add salt, egg, and rosemary. Combine everything carefully.
5. Get two pieces of parchment paper and put the pizza base in between them.
6. Roll it out with a rolling pin and try to make a circular shape. Peel off the parchment paper on top.
7. Get a fork and make several tiny holes in the pizza base.
8. Put the pizza base (bottom parchment paper still intact) on a baking tray and bake at 425°F for 10 to 16 minutes.
9. Remove the pizza base from the oven and start spreading the toppings on top. Finish off with crumbled feta.
10. Pop it in the oven once more using the same temperature and bake for 6 to 7 minutes.
11. Serve and enjoy.

# Veggies and Cottage Cheese Dip

**Instructions:**

- 1/2 cup baby carrots, blanched
- 1/2 cup snow peas, blanched
- 1/4 tsp lemon pepper
- 1/2 cup cottage cheese, low-fat

**Ingredients:**

1. Put all cottage cheese and lemon pepper in a bowl. Mix well.
2. Arrange the baby carrots, and peas, and dip on a platter. Serve.
3. You can also replace the carrots and peas with different vegetables.

# Fruit and Dark Greens Salad

**Ingredients:**

- 1 cup watermelon
- 1 cup cucumber sliced or spiral
- 1/2 cup raspberries
- 1 sliced avocado
- 1 cup baby broccoli
- 1 cup papaya
- 1/2 cup toasted almonds
- 4 cups baby kale

Dressing:

- 1/2 cup olive oil
- 1/2 cup master tonic
- 1/4 cup goji berries
- 4 dates
- a pinch of sea salt
- Tonic:
- 1/4 cup garlic, minced
- 1/4 cup onion, chopped
- 2 tbsp. horseradish, minced
- 2 knobs of turmeric, chopped
- 1 jalapeno pepper, chopped
- 32 oz. organic apple cider vinegar
- 1/4 cup fresh ginger, chopped
- juice of 1 lemon

**Instructions:**

1. Mix all salad ingredients except almonds.
2. Toss salad.

To make the dressing:

3. Mix master tonic, olive oil, and salt together.
4. In a blender, blend goji berries and dates until smooth.
5. Upon serving the salad, drizzle the dressing on, and gently add almonds.

To make the master tonic:

6. Add all ingredients to apple cider vinegar.
7. Blend all ingredients until everything is mixed well.
8. Let tonic sit in a jar for 1 to 2 weeks, shaking periodically.
9. Strain first before adding the leftover vinegar mixture into a jar with a cover.

# Grenade Salad

**Ingredients:**

- 4 cups arugula
- 1 large avocado
- 1/2 cup sliced fennel
- 1/2 cup sliced Anjou pears
- 1/4 cup pomegranate seeds

**Instructions:**

1. Mix all the ingredients except for the pomegranate seeds.
2. After mixing well, add the seeds. Mix again.
3. Serve with any type of desired dressing.

# Quinoa-based Asian Salad

**Ingredients:**

- 2 cups uncooked quinoa
- 4 cups vegetable broth
- 1 cup edamame
- 1/4 cup green onion, chopped
- 1-1/2 tsp. fresh mint, chopped
- 1/2 cup carrot, chopped
- 1/8 tsp. pepper flakes
- 1/2 tsp. orange zest, grated
- 2 tbsp. fresh Thai basil, chopped
- juice from half an orange
- 1 tsp. sesame seeds
- 1 tsp. sesame oil
- 1 tbsp. olive oil
- 1/8 tsp. black pepper

**Instructions:**

1. Mix the broth and quinoa in a pan.
2. Set the stove to high. Place the pan.
3. Let the mixture heat up for 12 to 14 minutes.
4. After heating, cover the pan and wait for 4 minutes.
5. Place the mixture in a separate container. Add in the rest of the ingredients.
6. Let it cool down before serving.

# Orange-Walnut Salad

**Ingredients:**

- 2 cups romaine lettuce, chopped coarsely
- 1 cucumber, peeled and deseeded, quartered lengthwise and chopped
- 1 cup arugula
- 2 navel oranges, peeled and chopped
- 1/4 cup red onion, sliced thinly
- 1 tbsp. walnut oil
- 2 tbsp. walnuts, chopped
- 1 tbsp. red wine vinegar
- 2 oz. blue cheese, gluten-free

**Instructions:**

1. In a salad bowl, carefully place the ingredients into layers.
2. Sprinkle with walnut oil and vinegar and toss.
3. With your hands, crumble blue cheese on top.
4. Serve immediately and enjoy.

# Chicken Salad Broccoli with Olive Oil

**Ingredients:**

- chicken breast
- broccoli
- olive oil
- mayonnaise or cream cheese
- Optional: onion

**Instructions:**

1. Steam a portion of chicken breast. Make sure it's just the right amount for your salad.
2. Once cooked, cut it into thin strips and set aside.
3. Briefly steam broccoli, make sure to not overcook them.
4. Mix the steamed chicken with the broccoli.
5. Add a little mayonnaise or cream.
6. Add olive oil.
7. Optional: add onion for added taste.

# Cobb and Egg Salad

**Ingredients:**

- 1 hard-boiled egg
- 3 oz. skinless, boneless chicken
- 1/4 cup cherry tomatoes
- 1 slice turkey bacon, crumbled
- feta cheese, crumbled
- bibb lettuce
- romaine lettuce
- lemon juice
- extra-virgin olive oil
- herbs of your choice

**Instruction:**

1. Make the salad dressing with lemon juice, extra-virgin olive oil, and herbs. Set aside.
2. Combine the solid ingredients in a large salad bowl.
3. Pour the dressing and toss to coat the salad.
4. Serve immediately.

# Asian Stir-Fry

**Ingredients:**

- 1 lb. beef or chicken, sliced
- 1/2 tsp. garlic powder
- 3/4 tsp. ground ginger
- 2 lb. stir-fry vegetables, chopped
- 1/4 cup apple cider vinegar
- 1/2 tsp. sea salt
- 1/8 cup honey
- 1 cup broth
- 6 tbsp. coconut aminos

**Instructions:**

1. In a stock pot over high heat, put and mix all the ingredients.
2. Bring to a boil. Then, lower the heat down to medium.
3. Cover the pot and allow the mixture to simmer for 20 minutes, or until the meat has cooked through and the vegetables are sufficiently tender.
4. Serve while hot.

# Horseradish Aioli and Roast Beef Sandwich

**Ingredients:**

- 1 tbsp. low-fat, less sodium Italian dressing
- 2 oz. roast beef, sliced
- 2 tbsp. reduced-fat mayonnaise
- 1 small cucumber, sliced
- 2 slices rye bread
- 1/2 cup fresh spinach
- 2 tsp. prepared horseradish

**Instructions:**

1. In a small bowl, combine horseradish and mayonnaise and stir well.
2. Put some mayonnaise mixture on each slice of bread.
3. Arrange the roast beef slices and spinach on one slice of bread and top it with the other slice of bread.
4. Serve the sandwich with slices of cucumber with dressing.

# Kale, Lentils, and Onion Pasta

**Ingredients:**

- 2-1/2 cups vegetable broth
- 3/4 cup dry lentils
- 1 tsp. salt
- 1 bay leaf
- 1/4 cup olive oil
- 1 large red onion, chopped
- 1 tsp. chopped fresh thyme
- 1/2 tsp. chopped fresh oregano
- 1/2 tsp. black pepper
- 1 bunch kale, stems removed and leaves coarsely chopped
- 1 pack of rotini pasta

**Instructions:**

1. In a saucepan, boil over high heat the following: vegetable broth, lentils, half teaspoon salt, and bay leaf.
2. Simmer down the heat to medium-low, cover, and then cook until the lentils are tender for about 20 minutes.
3. Add additional broth to keep the lentils moist if needed.
4. Discard the bay leaf once done.
5. As the lentils simmer, heat the olive oil in a skillet over medium-high heat.

6. Stir in the onion, thyme, oregano, pepper, and remaining salt. Stir-cook for a minute and add the sausage.
7. Reduce the heat to medium-low, and cook for 10 minutes.
8. Boil lightly salted water in a large pot over high heat.
9. Put in the kale and rotini pasta. Cook for 8 minutes until the rotini is firm.
10. Remove some of the cooking water, and set aside.
11. Drain pasta then return to the pot.
12. Stir in the lentils and onion mixture.
13. Using the reserved cooking liquid, adjust the dish's moistness according to your preference.
14. Sprinkle with nutritional yeast to serve.

# Barley and Chicken Soup

**Ingredients:**

- 4 cups vegetable broth
- 4 cups chicken broth
- 2-1/2 lb. chicken breast, bone and skin removed, cubed
- 2 cups butternut squash, peeled and cubed
- 2 cups yellow summer squash
- 2 cups cubed zucchini squash
- 1 cup white onion, diced
- 1 cup broccoli florets
- 8 oz. fresh mushrooms, chopped
- 1 cup barley
- 2 cups water
- 1 tbsp. garlic, minced
- 1 whole bay leaf
- 1/4 tsp. sea salt
- 1/4 tsp. ground black pepper

**Instructions:**

1. Pour the water, vegetable broth, and chicken broth in a large pot.
2. Add the chicken cubes, onion, garlic, bay leaf, salt, and black pepper.
3. Using medium-high heat, bring the contents of the pot to a boil.
4. Reduce the heat to low. Simmer for an hour.

5. Add the barley, broccoli, butternut squash, yellow summer squash, zucchini, and mushrooms into the pot.
6. Bring back to a boil.
7. Lower it to a simmer for about 60 to 120 minutes, or until vegetables have achieved your desired texture.
8. Transfer into a serving bowl immediately.

# Chia Seed and Strawberry Pudding

**Ingredients:**

- 1 cup strawberries, thinly sliced
- 3 tbsp. chia seeds
- 1 cup soy beverage, unsweetened and fortified

**Instructions:**

1. To create pudding, combine the soy beverage and chia seeds.
2. Refrigerate the mixture for half an hour. Stir the mixture every 5 minutes to prevent the chia seeds from sticking together.
3. As an alternative, blend the soy beverage and chia seeds in a food processor and let it chill in the refrigerator.
4. Slice strawberries lengthwise.
5. Pour chilled pudding into 2 glasses. Place the strawberry slices on top.
6. Serve and enjoy your pudding.

# Strawberry Smoothie

**Ingredients:**

- strawberries, 10pcs.
- banana slices
- orange juice, around 100 ml

**Instructions:**

1. Put all the ingredients in a blender.
2. Grind them until smooth.
3. Put it in a glass.

# Poached Egg Mytilene

**Ingredients:**

- lemon juice
- 1 tbsp. extra virgin olive oil
- 1-1/2 cups water
- 1-1/2 tbsp. white vinegar
- 2 eggs
- ground black pepper

**Instructions:**

1. Mix lemon juice and oil in a bowl and whisk until perfectly combined.
2. On a medium-sized pan, add water and vinegar. Let it boil slowly. Lower the heat.
3. Crack an egg, slowly letting it slip down the simmering water. Make sure not to break the egg yolk. Repeat the process on the other egg.
4. Allow eggs to cook for 2 to 3 minutes until the whites are firm and the yolks are slightly cooked outside and liquid inside.
5. Get them out of the water and place them on a plate.
6. Break the yolk and sprinkle the lemon juice mixture. Season with pepper.

# Veggie Omelet and Avocado Shake

**Ingredients:**

- 2 pcs. eggs
- cauliflower
- olive oil
- avocado
- ice

**Instructions:**

1. Scramble the eggs.
2. Use the leftover cauliflower.
3. If desired, you can sauté first the cauliflower in olive oil.
4. Pour in the scrambled eggs, but don't overcook your omelet.
5. Transfer on a nice plate.
6. To make the shake, cut fresh avocado in half and toss it in the blender along with ice. Blend well.
7. Serve on a tall glass with a straw.

# Bean Soup and Greens

**Ingredients:**

- 3 garlic cloves, minced
- 1 onion, diced
- 1 tbsp. coconut oil
- 2 tsp. freshly grated ginger
- 1 tsp. allspice
- 1 tsp. dried thyme
- 1-2 pcs. habanero or Scotch bonnet peppers, minced
- 1/2 tsp. black pepper
- 1/2 tsp. ground cinnamon
- 2 cups vegetable broth
- 14 oz.-can fire roasted tomatoes
- 14 oz.-can light coconut milk
- 14 oz.-can black beans, drained and rinsed
- 2 cans 14 oz. red kidney beans, drained and rinsed
- 2 tbsp. lime juice
- 1 lb. collard greens, destemmed and torn into 1-2-inch pieces

**Instructions:**

1. In a pot over medium heat, heat the coconut for about a minute or two.
2. Add onion and cook for about 5 minutes. Stir until soft and translucent.

3. Stir in the ginger, garlic, and pepper. Cook for another minute until fragrant.
4. Add in the thyme, black pepper, allspice, and cinnamon. Stir.
5. Pour in the broth and coconut milk, followed by the beans and tomatoes.
6. Adjust the heat to high and leave the soup to boil.
7. Reduce the heat for simmering without the cover, until the beans soften, about 10 minutes.
8. To make a thicker soup, blend a small amount of the soup using a conventional or immersion blender.
9. Throw in the collard greens upon serving.
10. Let it simmer for about 20 minutes, or until the greens are wilted and soft.
11. Remove the pot from the heat, then put the lime juice. Serve while hot.

# A 2-Week Plan to Start Managing Adult Scoliosis

Managing adult scoliosis is not impossible. It may be challenging, but with proper methods to follow, you can do it. Here is a sample 2-week plan to start managing your adult scoliosis.

## Week 1

For the first week, focus more on finding ways to adjust to doing activities that will help with your condition. For some, this will require major changes in their lifestyles that might affect even their routines. Doing the right routines will definitely be beneficial, especially in the long run.

Consult with your doctor to talk about your plans to change your diet, do some exercises, and do therapy. This way, your doctor can help you with these adjustments. At the same time, you can also worry less about how these changes may affect you especially if you have other conditions that also need to be looked into.

It's important to sort of treat this like changing your lifestyle to help yourself feel better.

**Diet**

In starting your diet, make sure that you try to get rid of the food items you need to avoid. This way, you can avoid getting tempted to either consume or use them in your meals. If you don't live alone, allot a cabinet where you can store all the ingredients you'll need, while the rest shall be stored separately. This need not be done in one go, especially if you're someone who doesn't have the means to just change everything in your pantry.

In addition to that, create a weekly meal plan, so you can prepare beforehand what you want to eat. Doing so will also help you with your groceries beforehand, which may also help with planning your budget. If you're cooking for your own, heating leftovers can also help with managing your budget and resources. While you may find meal plans that are catered for one sitting, you are free to modify them according to your preference.

Another tip is to do the transition gradually. There are two ways to start this—either by starting one healthy meal a day or assigning specific diet days for a week until you get used to this diet plan. That way, you can slowly adjust to the changes in your diet, as well as the new routine of being conscious in preparing your meals.

You may start by assigning three days a week to consume only healthy foods. In the following week, make it four days a week, until you're able to transition to eating healthy food for the whole week.

The goal of this first week is to motivate you to start living a healthier lifestyle by nourishing your body with proper nutrients instead of just eating what you want and what you are used to.

This will also be great if you don't have the capacity to throw away the food you currently have in your pantry. At least, this way, instead of wasting food items included in your do-not-consume list by throwing them away, you can just use them all up and replenish your supplies with the ingredients that are included in your must-have list. Just make sure that before you do, consult this with your doctor and/or dietitian first so they are informed that you are starting the diet gradually.

Additionally, you can also try to start some sort of a food journal or diary. You can take note of the food you eat every meal and how it affects you, if any. Then, as you transition to eating more of what's on your must-consume list, you might be able to see improvement along the way. However, take note that this is only the first week, so things may not improve at once.

**Therapy**

Starting therapy may seem like a daunting task, but keep in mind that you'll be doing it to help yourself. Keep open communication with your therapist throughout the program, from the consultation all the way through the therapy sessions, so that your therapist knows how the program helps and if it needs tweaking.

It is always best to start by learning about the different therapies that are ideal for those with adult scoliosis. As the second chapter discussed previously, there are quite a few you can check out to see if these would suit your needs and preferences. Make sure that you discuss this with your doctor or therapist before you do it.

For week 1, just make sure that you prep for it, especially before your scheduled therapy. Make sure that you are well rested, wearing proper clothes, and have done other things needed your doctor or therapist may require before the therapy. Take note also of what you need to remember after the therapy as there might be some things you need to do or avoid as post-therapy care.

**Exercise**

While it's highly recommended that you exercise, it's always better to consult first with your therapist and/or doctor before you start following an exercise routine. Talk to your therapist and your doctor about what types of exercises could be beneficial to you, which will not reverse the effects of the therapy you're getting. Keep in mind also that even low-intensity exercises can be beneficial, as long as they're done properly and regularly.

For week 1, do not hesitate to take your time to start exercising, especially if this is not something you are used to. As suggested in one of the previous chapters, you can try out yoga and swimming, but consult with your doctor first. On the other hand, if you're used to an active lifestyle, make sure that you still consult with your doctor if you're about to start a different workout routine. Try to stick to low-intensity exercises as much as possible.

## Week 2

For this week, you should be able to at least be familiar with the routine you've started with in week one. If you experienced no issues with any of them, then it's a good thing. However, if there are things that you have issues with any of the routines, make sure that you tell your doctor and therapist about these issues so that they can help you tweak what must be changed to help it become more efficient.

While it may not be that long, one week of implementing these changes in your diet and routine will definitely have a huge impact on you. Keeping a diary or journal may help you keep track of these important changes in your body and even your mood.

**Diet**

Continue what you have started during the first week. If you decide to transition with your diet slowly, then this is the time for you to try eating healthy for an entire week. While it may seem daunting, you may experience its benefits and improvements in your overall health.

Stick to the meal plan you make. Remember, you can repeat the meals you prepared to save time and budget. Keep looking for other recipes as well to spice up your meals.

If until this time, you still have food items in your pantry that you need to eliminate from your diet and want to get rid of, you can opt to not use them anymore—perhaps give them away to family or friends! Stick to your diet routine that you started on week 1 to achieve a much more beneficial result.

**Therapy**

After a week of trying out the therapy of your choice or recommended to you, you probably have additional notes regarding it. You can either continue the therapy program if you find it helpful, and make necessary changes with your therapist depending on how the therapy went during the first week.

Hopefully, changing your therapy won't be necessary in the second week as it would be much more ideal for that to happen in the first week. Unless the therapy is done not more than once or twice per week. Nonetheless, if you need to change your therapy, make sure you consult your doctor and/or therapist about it.

Keep writing in your journal about the changes and development, and even difficulties, you may be experiencing in your therapy sessions for the first week. This will be very helpful later on when your doctor and/or therapist checks on you eventually.

**Exercise**

Week 2 is obviously a continuation of what you have started on the first week, but that doesn't mean things need not change.

If in case you experience difficulty during your workout, stop doing it and take some rest. If necessary, contact your doctor or therapist to let them know what happened. Remember also that it's important to get the proper nutrition as you do these therapies and exercises.

However, if you find that the exercises you started are beneficial for you, then keep doing them. Just don't overdo them and give your body enough time to rest and recover from the exercise.

# Conclusion

## Final Thoughts on Managing Adult Scoliosis

Thank you for reading this guide on managing adult scoliosis. Making it through a detailed resource like this shows your commitment to taking control of your health, and that's truly inspiring. Living with scoliosis can bring challenges, but you've already taken the first step by arming yourself with knowledge—and that's something to be proud of.

When managing scoliosis, remember that small, consistent steps often lead to the best results. You don't need to overhaul your life overnight. Adjusting your diet, incorporating light exercise, and exploring therapy options, even one at a time, can all create positive change. Every effort you make, no matter how small it seems, brings you closer to feeling better and living more comfortably.

It's important to remind yourself that you're not alone in this. Many people face scoliosis and have found ways to live fulfilling lives. Surrounding yourself with supportive family, friends, and professionals can make all the difference. Don't hesitate to reach out to online communities or local groups—we all need encouragement. Sharing your experiences or hearing from others who truly understand can be a significant source of comfort and strength.

If you feel overwhelmed at times, that's okay. Scoliosis is a lifelong condition that takes patience to manage. Your body is unique, so what works for one person might not work for you. Be open to trying new therapies or making adjustments along the way with the guidance of healthcare professionals. Celebrate small victories, like discovering a routine that reduces pain or finding a new food that supports your health. These moments of progress add up and will keep you motivated.

One of the central themes of this guide is the power of balance—literally and figuratively. While managing scoliosis requires physical balance through posture and movement, it also calls for mental and emotional balance. Staying hopeful, allowing yourself time to rest, and knowing when to push forward or pause are all part of the process.

Diet, therapy, and exercise together form a strong foundation for managing your condition. By fueling your body with nutrient-rich foods, keeping your muscles active, and exploring therapies that suit your needs, you are equipping yourself with powerful tools. Remember, always consult with healthcare professionals to tailor these strategies specifically for your body's needs. Their expertise is key to keeping you on the right track and avoiding unnecessary risks.

Most importantly, don't give up on yourself. Your scoliosis is a part of your story, but it doesn't define who you are. You are capable of adapting, improving, and thriving. When setbacks occur, remind yourself how far you've come and the effort you've already invested in your health. Challenges may still arise, but now you have more understanding of how to face them.

Thank you for completing this guide. You have the knowledge, the tools, and the strength to move forward. Take this as the beginning of a healthier and more fulfilling chapter of your life. You've got this!

# FAQs

**What foods should I prioritize in my diet to help manage adult scoliosis?**

Focus on foods rich in calcium and vitamin D like leafy greens, milk, salmon, and eggs to strengthen bones. Include fruits, vegetables, and healthy fats such as nuts and avocados to reduce inflammation. Avoid heavily processed foods, sugary drinks, and excessive caffeine, as they can hinder bone health and increase inflammation.

**Can exercise help improve my scoliosis?**

Yes! Low-impact exercises like yoga, swimming, and core-strengthening routines are beneficial. They help improve posture, strengthen muscles supporting the spine, and reduce discomfort. Always consult your doctor or therapist before starting a new exercise program to ensure it's safe for your specific condition.

**Is it okay to try chiropractic care for scoliosis?**

Chiropractic care can be helpful for managing scoliosis, especially for improving mobility and reducing muscle tension. Look for a chiropractor who specializes in scoliosis treatment and consult your doctor to ensure it complements your overall care plan.

**How can I make daily activities easier with scoliosis?**

Focus on ergonomics! Use chairs with proper lumbar support, sleep in positions that keep your spine aligned (like on your back with a pillow under your knees), and invest in tools like lumbar pillows or standing desks. Small adjustments in how you sit, stand, and move can make a significant difference in managing your discomfort.

**What are some signs that my scoliosis is progressing?**

Watch for increased back pain, fatigue, uneven shoulders or hips, and difficulty completing daily tasks. If you experience any of these, consult your healthcare provider as it may be time to reassess your treatment plan.

**How often should I consult a specialist when managing scoliosis?**

This depends on the severity of your condition, but regular checkups every 6 to 12 months are usually recommended. If you're starting new therapies or experiencing changes in your symptoms, schedule a visit sooner for updated guidance.

**Can emotional health be affected by scoliosis, and how do I improve it?**

Yes, scoliosis can impact confidence and emotional well-being due to pain or changes in appearance. Joining support groups, talking to a therapist, and practicing relaxation techniques like mindfulness can help. Celebrate your progress and focus on all the positive steps you're taking to manage your condition.

# References and Helpful Links

Scoliosis. (2025b, February 7). Cleveland Clinic. https://my.clevelandclinic.org/health/diseases/15837-adult-scoliosis

Erika. (2024, November 29). Best Diet for Scoliosis | Scoliosis SOS. Scoliosis SOS. https://www.scoliosissos.com/blog/best-diet-for-scoliosis/

Choi, S., Jo, H., Park, S., Sung, W., Keum, D., & Kim, E. (2020). The effectiveness and safety of acupuncture for scoliosis. Medicine, 99(50), e23238. https://doi.org/10.1097/md.0000000000023238

Nalda, T. (2024, March 19). Scoliosis and Diet: 4 foods to add to your grocery list. Scoliosis Reduction Center®. https://www.scoliosisreductioncenter.com/blog/scoliosis-and-diet-4-foods-to-add-to-your-grocery-list

ScoliSMART. (2025, February 18). Scoliosis Nutrition | Treating Scoliosis. Treating Scoliosis. https://www.treatingscoliosis.com/scoliosis-nutrition/

Scoliosis. (2025, February 7). Cleveland Clinic. https://my.clevelandclinic.org/health/diseases/15837-scoliosis

Schroth method for scoliosis. (2023, March 14). Johns Hopkins Medicine. https://www.hopkinsmedicine.org/health/conditions-and-diseases/scoliosis/schroth-method-for-scoliosis

Rladmin. (2022, December 5). Types of Scoliosis: Which One Do You Have? by EIH. Effective Integrative Healthcare LLC. https://www.eihmd.com/2020/01/21/types-of-scoliosis-which-one-do-you-have/

www.ingramcontent.com/pod-product-compliance
Lightning Source LLC
LaVergne TN
LVHW010403070526
838199LV00065B/5883